NAME:

DATE:

TIME START:

TIME END:

AF490496

WARM-UP	TIME	NOTES

STRETCH:	TIME	NOTES

EXERCISE:	SET 1		SET 2		SET 3		SET 4	
	REPS	WEIGHT	REPS	WEIGHT	REPS	WEIGHT	REPS	WEIGHT

CARDIO:	TIME	DISTANCE	PACE	HR

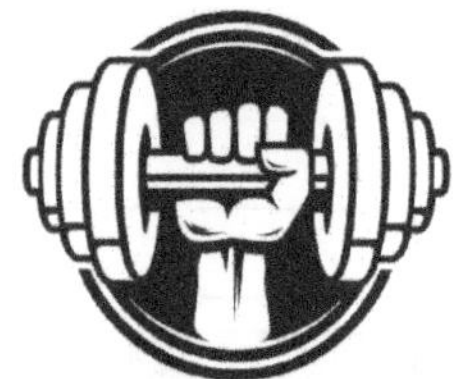

NAME:

DATE:

TIME START:

TIME END:

WARM-UP	TIME	NOTES

STRETCH:	TIME	NOTES

EXERCISE:	SET 1		SET 2		SET 3		SET 4	
	REPS	WEIGHT	REPS	WEIGHT	REPS	WEIGHT	REPS	WEIGHT

CARDIO:	TIME	DISTANCE	PACE	HR

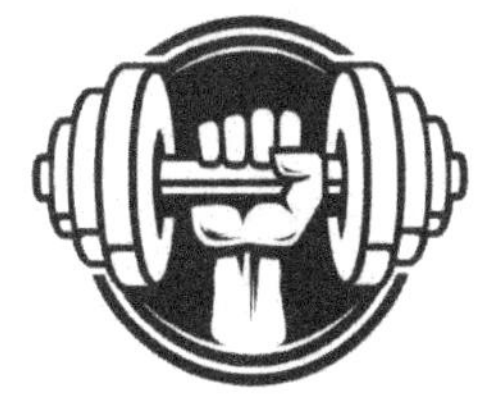

NAME:

DATE:

TIME START:

TIME END:

WARM-UP	TIME	NOTES

STRETCH:	TIME	NOTES

EXERCISE:	SET 1		SET 2		SET 3		SET 4	
	REPS	WEIGHT	REPS	WEIGHT	REPS	WEIGHT	REPS	WEIGHT

CARDIO:	TIME	DISTANCE	PACE	HR

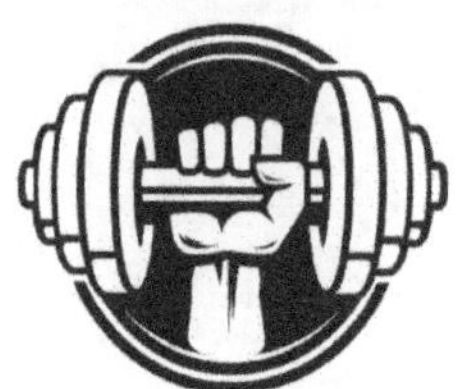

NAME: ___________________________

DATE: ___________________________

TIME START: ___________________________

TIME END: ___________________________

WARM-UP	TIME	NOTES

STRETCH:	TIME	NOTES

EXERCISE:	SET 1		SET 2		SET 3		SET 4	
	REPS	WEIGHT	REPS	WEIGHT	REPS	WEIGHT	REPS	WEIGHT

CARDIO:	TIME	DISTANCE	PACE	HR

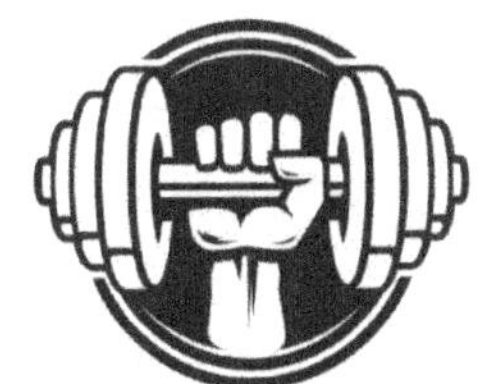

NAME: ___________________________

DATE: ___________________________

TIME START: _____________________

TIME END: _______________________

WARM-UP	TIME	NOTES

STRETCH:	TIME	NOTES

EXERCISE:	SET 1		SET 2		SET 3		SET 4	
	REPS	WEIGHT	REPS	WEIGHT	REPS	WEIGHT	REPS	WEIGHT

CARDIO:	TIME	DISTANCE	PACE	HR

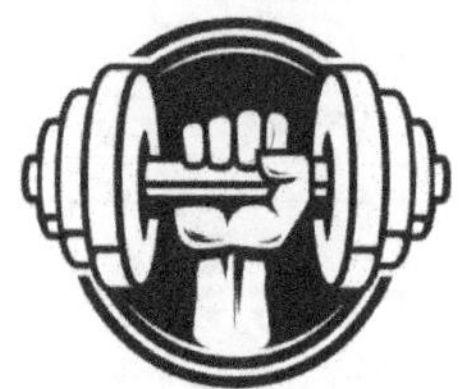

NAME:

DATE:

TIME START:

TIME END:

WARM-UP	TIME	NOTES

STRETCH:	TIME	NOTES

EXERCISE:	SET 1		SET 2		SET 3		SET 4	
	REPS	WEIGHT	REPS	WEIGHT	REPS	WEIGHT	REPS	WEIGHT

CARDIO:	TIME	DISTANCE	PACE	HR

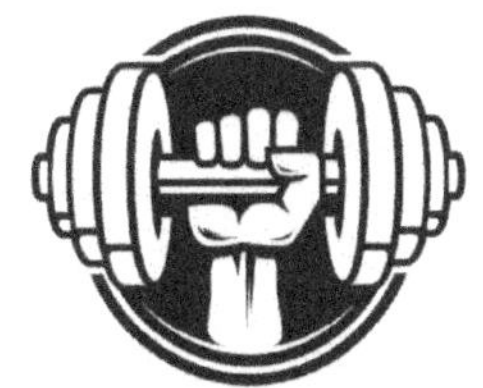

NAME:

DATE:

TIME START:

TIME END:

WARM-UP	TIME	NOTES

STRETCH:	TIME	NOTES

EXERCISE:	SET 1		SET 2		SET 3		SET 4	
	REPS	WEIGHT	REPS	WEIGHT	REPS	WEIGHT	REPS	WEIGHT

CARDIO:	TIME	DISTANCE	PACE	HR

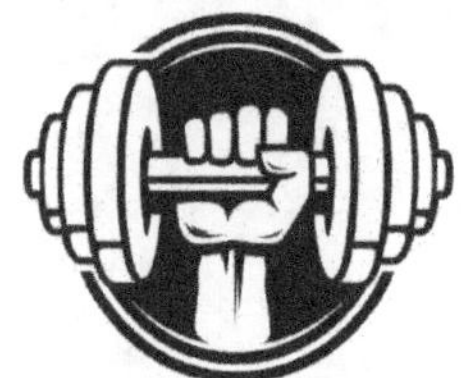

NAME:

DATE:

TIME START:

TIME END:

WARM-UP	TIME	NOTES

STRETCH:	TIME	NOTES

EXERCISE:	SET 1		SET 2		SET 3		SET 4	
	REPS	WEIGHT	REPS	WEIGHT	REPS	WEIGHT	REPS	WEIGHT

CARDIO:	TIME	DISTANCE	PACE	HR

NAME:

DATE:

TIME START:

TIME END:

WARM-UP	TIME	NOTES

STRETCH:	TIME	NOTES

EXERCISE:	SET 1		SET 2		SET 3		SET 4	
	REPS	WEIGHT	REPS	WEIGHT	REPS	WEIGHT	REPS	WEIGHT

CARDIO:	TIME	DISTANCE	PACE	HR

NAME:

DATE:

TIME START:

TIME END:

WARM-UP	TIME	NOTES

STRETCH:	TIME	NOTES

EXERCISE:	SET 1		SET 2		SET 3		SET 4	
	REPS	WEIGHT	REPS	WEIGHT	REPS	WEIGHT	REPS	WEIGHT

CARDIO:	TIME	DISTANCE	PACE	HR

NAME: ______________________

DATE: ______________________

TIME START: ______________________

TIME END: ______________________

WARM-UP	TIME	NOTES

STRETCH:	TIME	NOTES

EXERCISE:	SET 1		SET 2		SET 3		SET 4	
	REPS	WEIGHT	REPS	WEIGHT	REPS	WEIGHT	REPS	WEIGHT

CARDIO:	TIME	DISTANCE	PACE	HR

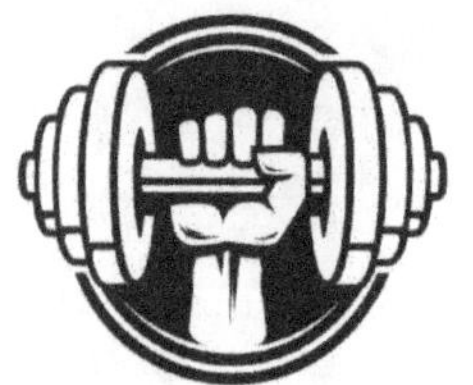

NAME:

DATE:

TIME START:

TIME END:

WARM-UP	TIME	NOTES

STRETCH:	TIME	NOTES

EXERCISE:	SET 1		SET 2		SET 3		SET 4	
	REPS	WEIGHT	REPS	WEIGHT	REPS	WEIGHT	REPS	WEIGHT

CARDIO:	TIME	DISTANCE	PACE	HR

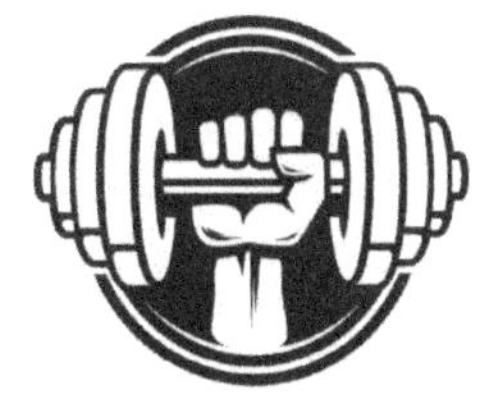

NAME: ______________________________

DATE: ______________________________

TIME START: ______________________________

TIME END: ______________________________

WARM-UP	TIME	NOTES

STRETCH:	TIME	NOTES

EXERCISE:	SET 1		SET 2		SET 3		SET 4	
	REPS	WEIGHT	REPS	WEIGHT	REPS	WEIGHT	REPS	WEIGHT

CARDIO:	TIME	DISTANCE	PACE	HR

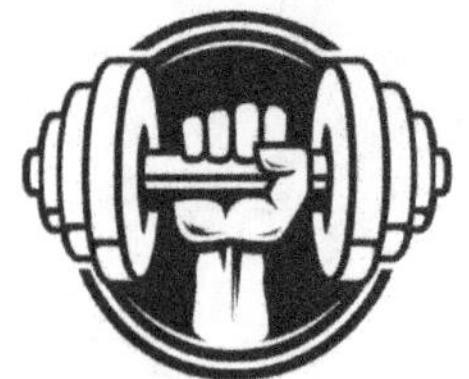

NAME:	
DATE:	
TIME START:	
TIME END:	

WARM-UP	TIME	NOTES

STRETCH:	TIME	NOTES

EXERCISE:	SET 1		SET 2		SET 3		SET 4	
	REPS	WEIGHT	REPS	WEIGHT	REPS	WEIGHT	REPS	WEIGHT

CARDIO:	TIME	DISTANCE	PACE	HR

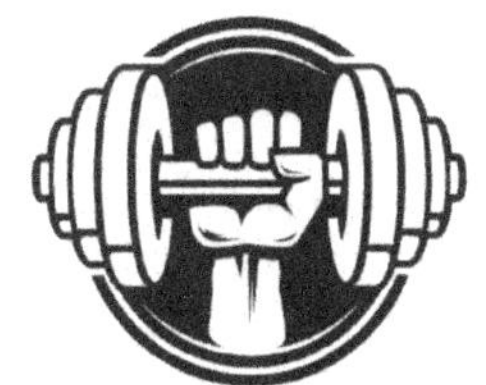

NAME:

DATE:

TIME START:

TIME END:

WARM-UP	TIME	NOTES

STRETCH:	TIME	NOTES

EXERCISE:	SET 1		SET 2		SET 3		SET 4	
	REPS	WEIGHT	REPS	WEIGHT	REPS	WEIGHT	REPS	WEIGHT

CARDIO:	TIME	DISTANCE	PACE	HR

NAME:_______________________

DATE:_______________________

TIME START:_______________________

TIME END:_______________________

WARM-UP	TIME	NOTES

STRETCH:	TIME	NOTES

EXERCISE:	SET 1		SET 2		SET 3		SET 4	
	REPS	WEIGHT	REPS	WEIGHT	REPS	WEIGHT	REPS	WEIGHT

CARDIO:	TIME	DISTANCE	PACE	HR

NAME: _______________

DATE: _______________

TIME START: _______________

TIME END: _______________

WARM-UP	TIME	NOTES

STRETCH:	TIME	NOTES

EXERCISE:	SET 1		SET 2		SET 3		SET 4	
	REPS	WEIGHT	REPS	WEIGHT	REPS	WEIGHT	REPS	WEIGHT

CARDIO:	TIME	DISTANCE	PACE	HR

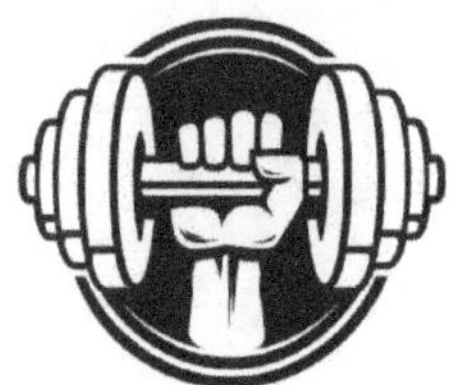

NAME: _______________

DATE: _______________

TIME START: _______________

TIME END: _______________

WARM-UP	TIME	NOTES

STRETCH:	TIME	NOTES

EXERCISE:	SET 1		SET 2		SET 3		SET 4	
	REPS	WEIGHT	REPS	WEIGHT	REPS	WEIGHT	REPS	WEIGHT

CARDIO:	TIME	DISTANCE	PACE	HR

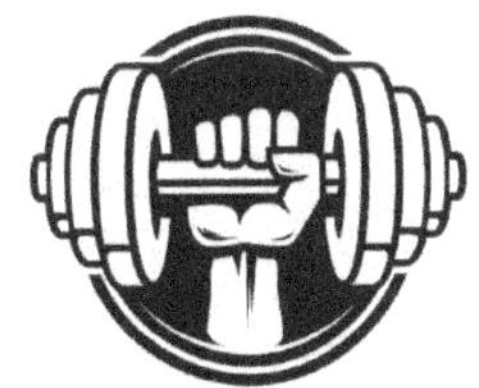

NAME:

DATE:

TIME START:

TIME END:

WARM-UP	TIME	NOTES

STRETCH:	TIME	NOTES

EXERCISE:	SET 1		SET 2		SET 3		SET 4	
	REPS	WEIGHT	REPS	WEIGHT	REPS	WEIGHT	REPS	WEIGHT

CARDIO:	TIME	DISTANCE	PACE	HR

NAME: ___________________

DATE: ___________________

TIME START: ___________________

TIME END: ___________________

WARM-UP	TIME	NOTES

STRETCH:	TIME	NOTES

EXERCISE:	SET 1		SET 2		SET 3		SET 4	
	REPS	WEIGHT	REPS	WEIGHT	REPS	WEIGHT	REPS	WEIGHT

CARDIO:	TIME	DISTANCE	PACE	HR

NAME:

DATE:

TIME START:

TIME END:

WARM-UP	TIME	NOTES

STRETCH:	TIME	NOTES

EXERCISE:	SET 1		SET 2		SET 3		SET 4	
	REPS	WEIGHT	REPS	WEIGHT	REPS	WEIGHT	REPS	WEIGHT

CARDIO:	TIME	DISTANCE	PACE	HR

NAME: _______________________

DATE: _______________________

TIME START: _______________________

TIME END: _______________________

WARM-UP	TIME	NOTES

STRETCH:	TIME	NOTES

EXERCISE:	SET 1		SET 2		SET 3		SET 4	
	REPS	WEIGHT	REPS	WEIGHT	REPS	WEIGHT	REPS	WEIGHT

CARDIO:	TIME	DISTANCE	PACE	HR

WARM-UP	TIME	NOTES

STRETCH:	TIME	NOTES

EXERCISE:	SET 1		SET 2		SET 3		SET 4	
	REPS	WEIGHT	REPS	WEIGHT	REPS	WEIGHT	REPS	WEIGHT

CARDIO:	TIME	DISTANCE	PACE	HR

NAME:

DATE:

TIME START:

TIME END:

WARM-UP	TIME	NOTES

STRETCH:	TIME	NOTES

EXERCISE:	SET 1		SET 2		SET 3		SET 4	
	REPS	WEIGHT	REPS	WEIGHT	REPS	WEIGHT	REPS	WEIGHT

CARDIO:	TIME	DISTANCE	PACE	HR

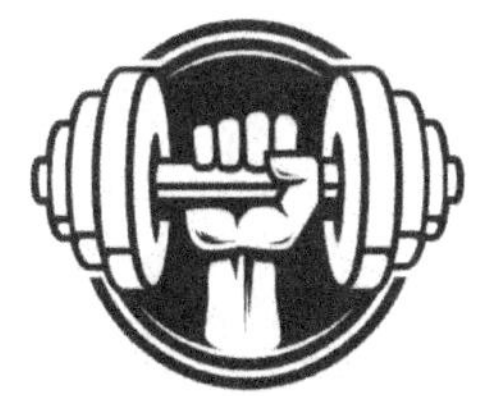

NAME:

DATE:

TIME START:

TIME END:

WARM-UP	TIME	NOTES

STRETCH:	TIME	NOTES

EXERCISE:	SET 1		SET 2		SET 3		SET 4	
	REPS	WEIGHT	REPS	WEIGHT	REPS	WEIGHT	REPS	WEIGHT

CARDIO:	TIME	DISTANCE	PACE	HR

NAME:

DATE:

TIME START:

TIME END:

WARM-UP	TIME	NOTES

STRETCH:	TIME	NOTES

EXERCISE:	SET 1		SET 2		SET 3		SET 4	
	REPS	WEIGHT	REPS	WEIGHT	REPS	WEIGHT	REPS	WEIGHT

CARDIO:	TIME	DISTANCE	PACE	HR

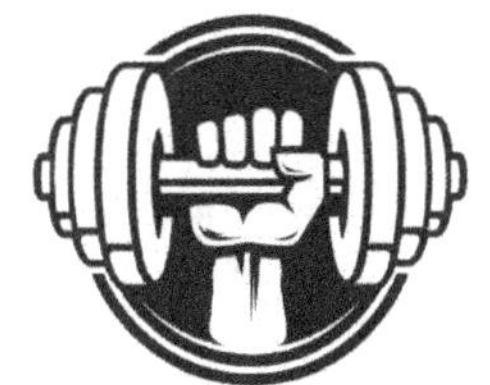

<table>
<tr><th>WARM-UP</th><th>TIME</th><th>NOTES</th></tr>
<tr><td></td><td></td><td></td></tr>
<tr><td></td><td></td><td></td></tr>
<tr><td></td><td></td><td></td></tr>
<tr><td></td><td></td><td></td></tr>
</table>

NAME:

DATE:

TIME START:

TIME END:

STRETCH:	TIME	NOTES

EXERCISE:	SET 1		SET 2		SET 3		SET 4	
	REPS	WEIGHT	REPS	WEIGHT	REPS	WEIGHT	REPS	WEIGHT

CARDIO:	TIME	DISTANCE	PACE	HR

NAME:

DATE:

TIME START:

TIME END:

WARM-UP	TIME	NOTES

STRETCH:	TIME	NOTES

EXERCISE:	SET 1		SET 2		SET 3		SET 4	
	REPS	WEIGHT	REPS	WEIGHT	REPS	WEIGHT	REPS	WEIGHT

CARDIO:	TIME	DISTANCE	PACE	HR

NAME:

DATE:

TIME START:

TIME END:

WARM-UP	TIME	NOTES

STRETCH:	TIME	NOTES

EXERCISE:	SET 1		SET 2		SET 3		SET 4	
	REPS	WEIGHT	REPS	WEIGHT	REPS	WEIGHT	REPS	WEIGHT

CARDIO:	TIME	DISTANCE	PACE	HR

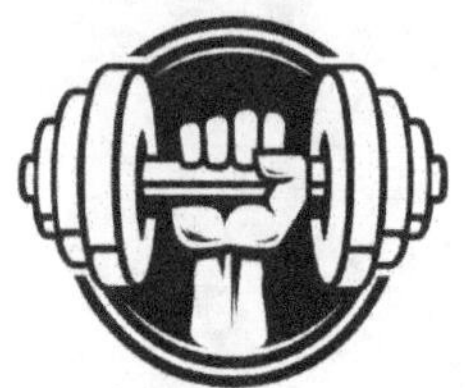

NAME:

DATE:

TIME START:

TIME END:

WARM-UP	TIME	NOTES

STRETCH:	TIME	NOTES

EXERCISE:	SET 1		SET 2		SET 3		SET 4	
	REPS	WEIGHT	REPS	WEIGHT	REPS	WEIGHT	REPS	WEIGHT

CARDIO:	TIME	DISTANCE	PACE	HR

NAME:

DATE:

TIME START:

TIME END:

WARM-UP	TIME	NOTES

STRETCH:	TIME	NOTES

EXERCISE:	SET 1		SET 2		SET 3		SET 4	
	REPS	WEIGHT	REPS	WEIGHT	REPS	WEIGHT	REPS	WEIGHT

CARDIO:	TIME	DISTANCE	PACE	HR

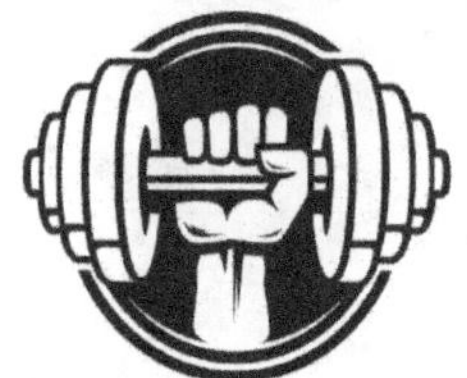

NAME:

DATE:

TIME START:

TIME END:

WARM-UP	TIME	NOTES

STRETCH:	TIME	NOTES

EXERCISE:	SET 1		SET 2		SET 3		SET 4	
	REPS	WEIGHT	REPS	WEIGHT	REPS	WEIGHT	REPS	WEIGHT

CARDIO:	TIME	DISTANCE	PACE	HR

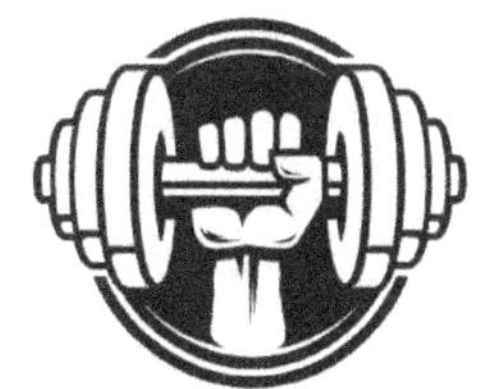

NAME:

DATE:

TIME START:

TIME END:

WARM-UP	TIME	NOTES

STRETCH:	TIME	NOTES

EXERCISE:	SET 1		SET 2		SET 3		SET 4	
	REPS	WEIGHT	REPS	WEIGHT	REPS	WEIGHT	REPS	WEIGHT

CARDIO:	TIME	DISTANCE	PACE	HR

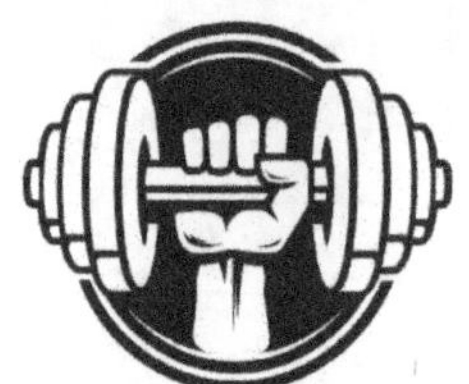

NAME:

DATE:

TIME START:

TIME END:

WARM-UP	TIME	NOTES

STRETCH:	TIME	NOTES

EXERCISE:	SET 1		SET 2		SET 3		SET 4	
	REPS	WEIGHT	REPS	WEIGHT	REPS	WEIGHT	REPS	WEIGHT

CARDIO:	TIME	DISTANCE	PACE	HR

NAME: _______________________

DATE: _______________________

TIME START: _______________________

TIME END: _______________________

WARM-UP	TIME	NOTES

STRETCH:	TIME	NOTES

EXERCISE:	SET 1		SET 2		SET 3		SET 4	
	REPS	WEIGHT	REPS	WEIGHT	REPS	WEIGHT	REPS	WEIGHT

CARDIO:	TIME	DISTANCE	PACE	HR

NAME:______________________

DATE:______________________

TIME START:______________________

TIME END:______________________

WARM-UP	TIME	NOTES

STRETCH:	TIME	NOTES

EXERCISE:	SET 1		SET 2		SET 3		SET 4	
	REPS	WEIGHT	REPS	WEIGHT	REPS	WEIGHT	REPS	WEIGHT

CARDIO:	TIME	DISTANCE	PACE	HR

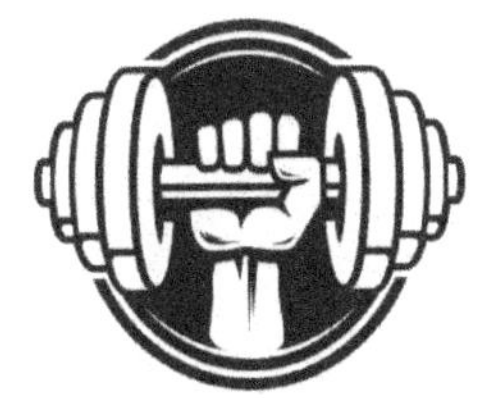

NAME:

DATE:

TIME START:

TIME END:

WARM-UP	TIME	NOTES

STRETCH:	TIME	NOTES

EXERCISE:	SET 1		SET 2		SET 3		SET 4	
	REPS	WEIGHT	REPS	WEIGHT	REPS	WEIGHT	REPS	WEIGHT

CARDIO:	TIME	DISTANCE	PACE	HR

NAME:

DATE:

TIME START:

TIME END:

WARM-UP	TIME	NOTES

STRETCH:	TIME	NOTES

EXERCISE:	SET 1		SET 2		SET 3		SET 4	
	REPS	WEIGHT	REPS	WEIGHT	REPS	WEIGHT	REPS	WEIGHT

CARDIO:	TIME	DISTANCE	PACE	HR

NAME:_______________________

DATE:_______________________

TIME START:_________________

TIME END:___________________

WARM-UP	TIME	NOTES

STRETCH:	TIME	NOTES

EXERCISE:	SET 1		SET 2		SET 3		SET 4	
	REPS	WEIGHT	REPS	WEIGHT	REPS	WEIGHT	REPS	WEIGHT

CARDIO:	TIME	DISTANCE	PACE	HR

NAME:

DATE:

TIME START:

TIME END:

WARM-UP	TIME	NOTES

STRETCH:	TIME	NOTES

EXERCISE:	SET 1		SET 2		SET 3		SET 4	
	REPS	WEIGHT	REPS	WEIGHT	REPS	WEIGHT	REPS	WEIGHT

CARDIO:	TIME	DISTANCE	PACE	HR

NAME:

DATE:

TIME START:

TIME END:

WARM-UP	TIME	NOTES

STRETCH:	TIME	NOTES

EXERCISE:	SET 1		SET 2		SET 3		SET 4	
	REPS	WEIGHT	REPS	WEIGHT	REPS	WEIGHT	REPS	WEIGHT

CARDIO:	TIME	DISTANCE	PACE	HR

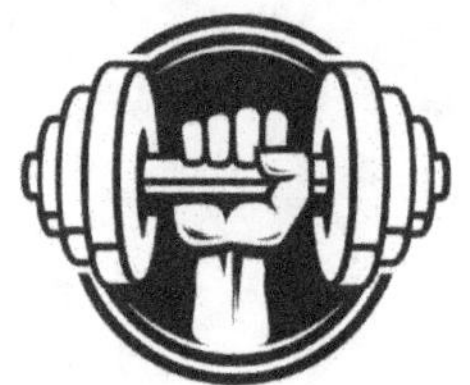

NAME:

DATE:

TIME START:

TIME END:

WARM-UP	TIME	NOTES

STRETCH:	TIME	NOTES

EXERCISE:	SET 1		SET 2		SET 3		SET 4	
	REPS	WEIGHT	REPS	WEIGHT	REPS	WEIGHT	REPS	WEIGHT

CARDIO:	TIME	DISTANCE	PACE	HR

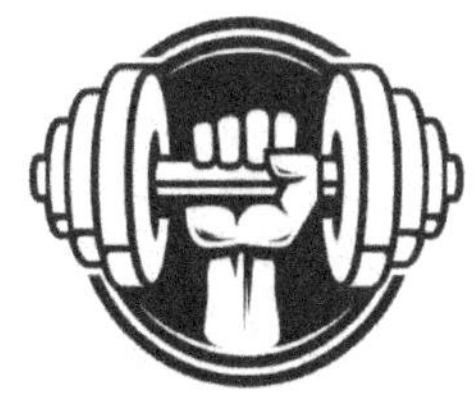

NAME:

DATE:

TIME START:

TIME END:

WARM-UP	TIME	NOTES

STRETCH:	TIME	NOTES

EXERCISE:	SET 1		SET 2		SET 3		SET 4	
	REPS	WEIGHT	REPS	WEIGHT	REPS	WEIGHT	REPS	WEIGHT

CARDIO:	TIME	DISTANCE	PACE	HR

NAME:_______________________________

DATE:_______________________________

TIME START:_______________________________

TIME END:_______________________________

WARM-UP	TIME	NOTES

STRETCH:	TIME	NOTES

EXERCISE:	SET 1		SET 2		SET 3		SET 4	
	REPS	WEIGHT	REPS	WEIGHT	REPS	WEIGHT	REPS	WEIGHT

CARDIO:	TIME	DISTANCE	PACE	HR

NAME:

DATE:

TIME START:

TIME END:

WARM-UP	TIME	NOTES

STRETCH:	TIME	NOTES

EXERCISE:	SET 1		SET 2		SET 3		SET 4	
	REPS	WEIGHT	REPS	WEIGHT	REPS	WEIGHT	REPS	WEIGHT

CARDIO:	TIME	DISTANCE	PACE	HR

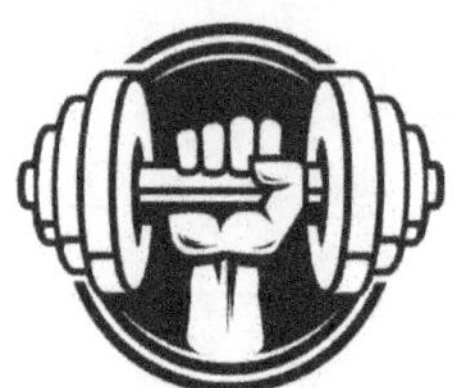

NAME: ___________________

DATE: ___________________

TIME START: ___________________

TIME END: ___________________

WARM-UP	TIME	NOTES

STRETCH:	TIME	NOTES

EXERCISE:	SET 1		SET 2		SET 3		SET 4	
	REPS	WEIGHT	REPS	WEIGHT	REPS	WEIGHT	REPS	WEIGHT

CARDIO:	TIME	DISTANCE	PACE	HR

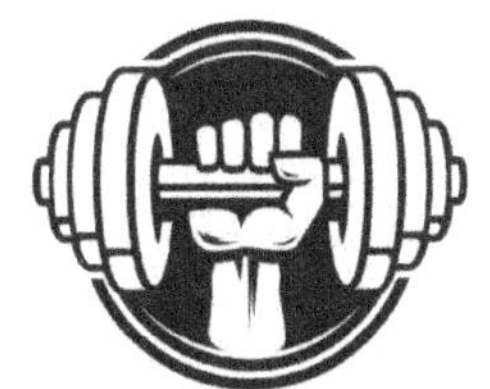

NAME:___________________________

DATE:___________________________

TIME START:___________________________

TIME END:___________________________

WARM-UP	TIME	NOTES

STRETCH:	TIME	NOTES

EXERCISE:	SET 1		SET 2		SET 3		SET 4	
	REPS	WEIGHT	REPS	WEIGHT	REPS	WEIGHT	REPS	WEIGHT

CARDIO:	TIME	DISTANCE	PACE	HR

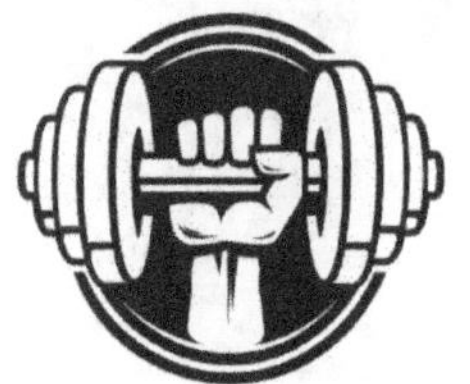

NAME:_______________________

DATE:_______________________

TIME START:_______________________

TIME END:_______________________

WARM-UP	TIME	NOTES

STRETCH:	TIME	NOTES

EXERCISE:	SET 1		SET 2		SET 3		SET 4	
	REPS	WEIGHT	REPS	WEIGHT	REPS	WEIGHT	REPS	WEIGHT

CARDIO:	TIME	DISTANCE	PACE	HR

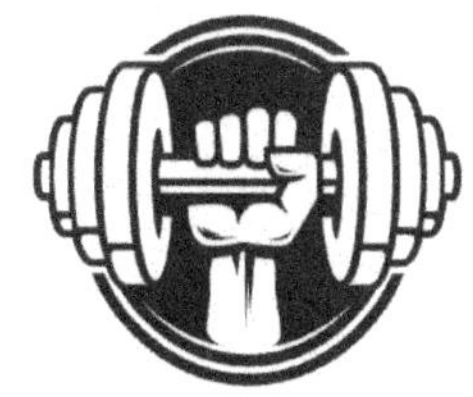

NAME: ___________

DATE: ___________

TIME START: ___________

TIME END: ___________

WARM-UP	TIME	NOTES

STRETCH:	TIME	NOTES

EXERCISE:	SET 1		SET 2		SET 3		SET 4	
	REPS	WEIGHT	REPS	WEIGHT	REPS	WEIGHT	REPS	WEIGHT

CARDIO:	TIME	DISTANCE	PACE	HR

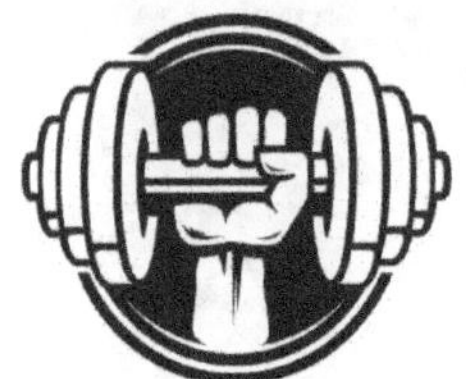

NAME:____________________

DATE:____________________

TIME START:____________________

TIME END:____________________

WARM-UP	TIME	NOTES

STRETCH:	TIME	NOTES

EXERCISE:	SET 1		SET 2		SET 3		SET 4	
	REPS	WEIGHT	REPS	WEIGHT	REPS	WEIGHT	REPS	WEIGHT

CARDIO:	TIME	DISTANCE	PACE	HR

NAME:

DATE:

TIME START:

TIME END:

WARM-UP	TIME	NOTES

STRETCH:	TIME	NOTES

EXERCISE:	SET 1		SET 2		SET 3		SET 4	
	REPS	WEIGHT	REPS	WEIGHT	REPS	WEIGHT	REPS	WEIGHT

CARDIO:	TIME	DISTANCE	PACE	HR

NAME:

DATE:

TIME START:

TIME END:

WARM-UP	TIME	NOTES

STRETCH:	TIME	NOTES

EXERCISE:	SET 1		SET 2		SET 3		SET 4	
	REPS	WEIGHT	REPS	WEIGHT	REPS	WEIGHT	REPS	WEIGHT

CARDIO:	TIME	DISTANCE	PACE	HR

NAME:

DATE:

TIME START:

TIME END:

WARM-UP	TIME	NOTES

STRETCH:	TIME	NOTES

EXERCISE:	SET 1		SET 2		SET 3		SET 4	
	REPS	WEIGHT	REPS	WEIGHT	REPS	WEIGHT	REPS	WEIGHT

CARDIO:	TIME	DISTANCE	PACE	HR

NAME:

DATE:

TIME START:

TIME END:

WARM-UP	TIME	NOTES

STRETCH:	TIME	NOTES

EXERCISE:	SET 1		SET 2		SET 3		SET 4	
	REPS	WEIGHT	REPS	WEIGHT	REPS	WEIGHT	REPS	WEIGHT

CARDIO:	TIME	DISTANCE	PACE	HR

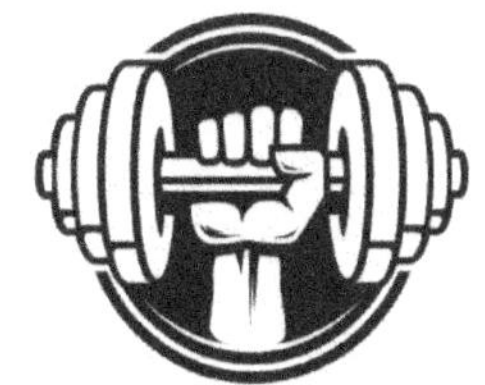

NAME:	
DATE:	
TIME START:	
TIME END:	

WARM-UP	TIME	NOTES

STRETCH:	TIME	NOTES

EXERCISE:	SET 1		SET 2		SET 3		SET 4	
	REPS	WEIGHT	REPS	WEIGHT	REPS	WEIGHT	REPS	WEIGHT

CARDIO:	TIME	DISTANCE	PACE	HR

NAME:

DATE:

TIME START:

TIME END:

WARM-UP	TIME	NOTES

STRETCH:	TIME	NOTES

EXERCISE:	SET 1		SET 2		SET 3		SET 4	
	REPS	WEIGHT	REPS	WEIGHT	REPS	WEIGHT	REPS	WEIGHT

CARDIO:	TIME	DISTANCE	PACE	HR

NAME:

DATE:

TIME START:

TIME END:

WARM-UP	TIME	NOTES

STRETCH:	TIME	NOTES

EXERCISE:	SET 1		SET 2		SET 3		SET 4	
	REPS	WEIGHT	REPS	WEIGHT	REPS	WEIGHT	REPS	WEIGHT

CARDIO:	TIME	DISTANCE	PACE	HR

NAME:

DATE:

TIME START:

TIME END:

WARM-UP	TIME	NOTES

STRETCH:	TIME	NOTES

EXERCISE:	SET 1		SET 2		SET 3		SET 4	
	REPS	WEIGHT	REPS	WEIGHT	REPS	WEIGHT	REPS	WEIGHT

CARDIO:	TIME	DISTANCE	PACE	HR

NAME:

DATE:

TIME START:

TIME END:

WARM-UP	TIME	NOTES

STRETCH:	TIME	NOTES

EXERCISE:	SET 1		SET 2		SET 3		SET 4	
	REPS	WEIGHT	REPS	WEIGHT	REPS	WEIGHT	REPS	WEIGHT

CARDIO:	TIME	DISTANCE	PACE	HR

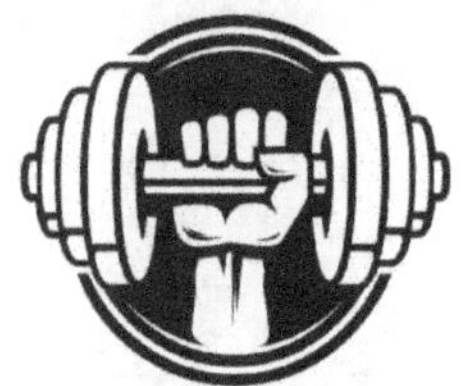

NAME:_______________________

DATE:_______________________

TIME START:_______________________

TIME END:_______________________

WARM-UP	TIME	NOTES

STRETCH:	TIME	NOTES

EXERCISE:	SET 1		SET 2		SET 3		SET 4	
	REPS	WEIGHT	REPS	WEIGHT	REPS	WEIGHT	REPS	WEIGHT

CARDIO:	TIME	DISTANCE	PACE	HR

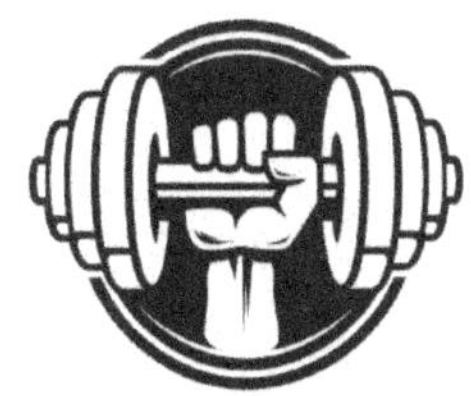

NAME:

DATE:

TIME START:

TIME END:

WARM-UP	TIME	NOTES

STRETCH:	TIME	NOTES

EXERCISE:	SET 1		SET 2		SET 3		SET 4	
	REPS	WEIGHT	REPS	WEIGHT	REPS	WEIGHT	REPS	WEIGHT

CARDIO:	TIME	DISTANCE	PACE	HR

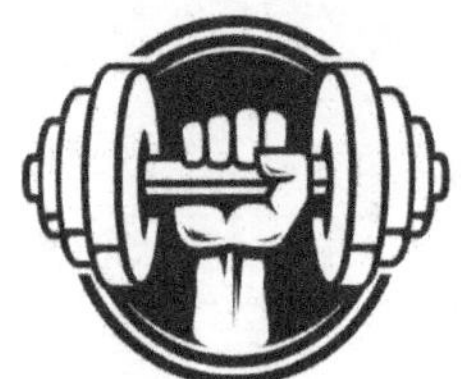

NAME:

DATE:

TIME START:

TIME END:

WARM-UP	TIME	NOTES

STRETCH:	TIME	NOTES

EXERCISE:	SET 1		SET 2		SET 3		SET 4	
	REPS	WEIGHT	REPS	WEIGHT	REPS	WEIGHT	REPS	WEIGHT

CARDIO:	TIME	DISTANCE	PACE	HR

NAME:

DATE:

TIME START:

TIME END:

WARM-UP	TIME	NOTES

STRETCH:	TIME	NOTES

EXERCISE:	SET 1		SET 2		SET 3		SET 4	
	REPS	WEIGHT	REPS	WEIGHT	REPS	WEIGHT	REPS	WEIGHT

CARDIO:	TIME	DISTANCE	PACE	HR

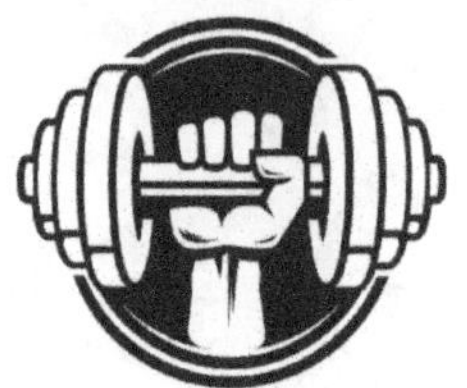

NAME:

DATE:

TIME START:

TIME END:

WARM-UP	TIME	NOTES

STRETCH:	TIME	NOTES

EXERCISE:	SET 1		SET 2		SET 3		SET 4	
	REPS	WEIGHT	REPS	WEIGHT	REPS	WEIGHT	REPS	WEIGHT

CARDIO:	TIME	DISTANCE	PACE	HR

NAME:	
DATE:	
TIME START:	
TIME END:	

WARM-UP	TIME	NOTES

STRETCH:	TIME	NOTES

EXERCISE:	SET 1		SET 2		SET 3		SET 4	
	REPS	WEIGHT	REPS	WEIGHT	REPS	WEIGHT	REPS	WEIGHT

CARDIO:	TIME	DISTANCE	PACE	HR

NAME:

DATE:

TIME START:

TIME END:

WARM-UP	TIME	NOTES

STRETCH:	TIME	NOTES

EXERCISE:	SET 1		SET 2		SET 3		SET 4	
	REPS	WEIGHT	REPS	WEIGHT	REPS	WEIGHT	REPS	WEIGHT

CARDIO:	TIME	DISTANCE	PACE	HR

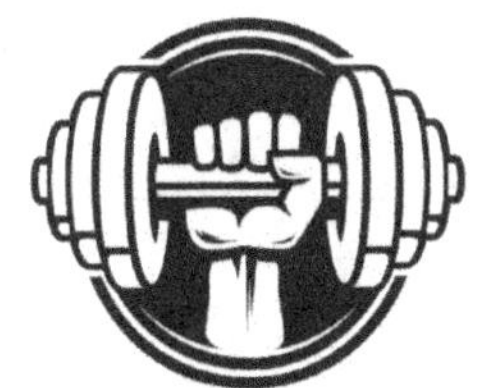

NAME: _______________________

DATE: _______________________

TIME START: _______________________

TIME END: _______________________

WARM-UP	TIME	NOTES

STRETCH:	TIME	NOTES

EXERCISE:	SET 1		SET 2		SET 3		SET 4	
	REPS	WEIGHT	REPS	WEIGHT	REPS	WEIGHT	REPS	WEIGHT

CARDIO:	TIME	DISTANCE	PACE	HR

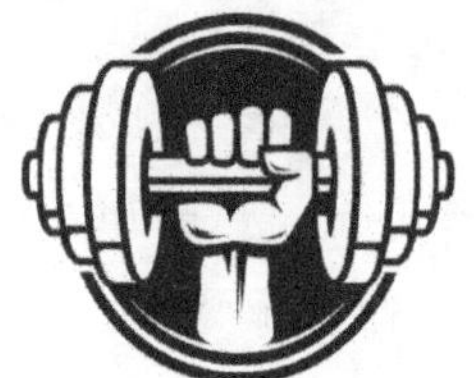

NAME:

DATE:

TIME START:

TIME END:

WARM-UP	TIME	NOTES

STRETCH:	TIME	NOTES

EXERCISE:	SET 1		SET 2		SET 3		SET 4	
	REPS	WEIGHT	REPS	WEIGHT	REPS	WEIGHT	REPS	WEIGHT

CARDIO:	TIME	DISTANCE	PACE	HR

NAME:

DATE:

TIME START:

TIME END:

WARM-UP	TIME	NOTES

STRETCH:	TIME	NOTES

EXERCISE:	SET 1		SET 2		SET 3		SET 4	
	REPS	WEIGHT	REPS	WEIGHT	REPS	WEIGHT	REPS	WEIGHT

CARDIO:	TIME	DISTANCE	PACE	HR

NAME:

DATE:

TIME START:

TIME END:

WARM-UP	TIME	NOTES

STRETCH:	TIME	NOTES

EXERCISE:	SET 1		SET 2		SET 3		SET 4	
	REPS	WEIGHT	REPS	WEIGHT	REPS	WEIGHT	REPS	WEIGHT

CARDIO:	TIME	DISTANCE	PACE	HR

NAME: _______________

DATE: _______________

TIME START: _______________

TIME END: _______________

WARM-UP	TIME	NOTES

STRETCH:	TIME	NOTES

EXERCISE:	SET 1		SET 2		SET 3		SET 4	
	REPS	WEIGHT	REPS	WEIGHT	REPS	WEIGHT	REPS	WEIGHT

CARDIO:	TIME	DISTANCE	PACE	HR

NAME:

DATE:

TIME START:

TIME END:

WARM-UP	TIME	NOTES

STRETCH:	TIME	NOTES

EXERCISE:	SET 1		SET 2		SET 3		SET 4	
	REPS	WEIGHT	REPS	WEIGHT	REPS	WEIGHT	REPS	WEIGHT

CARDIO:	TIME	DISTANCE	PACE	HR

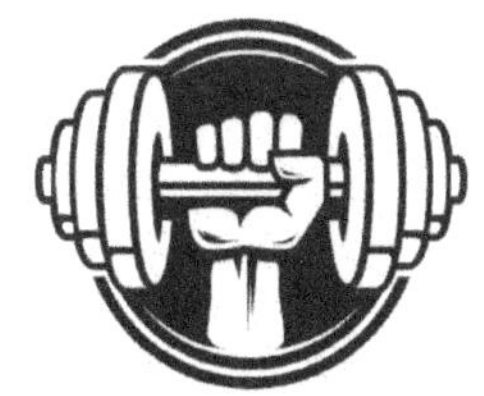

NAME:

DATE:

TIME START:

TIME END:

WARM-UP	TIME	NOTES

STRETCH:	TIME	NOTES

EXERCISE:	SET 1		SET 2		SET 3		SET 4	
	REPS	WEIGHT	REPS	WEIGHT	REPS	WEIGHT	REPS	WEIGHT

CARDIO:	TIME	DISTANCE	PACE	HR

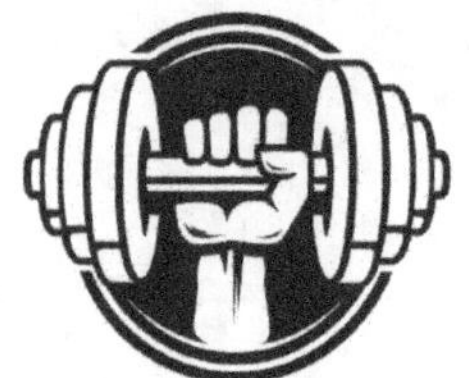

NAME:

DATE:

TIME START:

TIME END:

WARM-UP	TIME	NOTES

STRETCH:	TIME	NOTES

EXERCISE:	SET 1		SET 2		SET 3		SET 4	
	REPS	WEIGHT	REPS	WEIGHT	REPS	WEIGHT	REPS	WEIGHT

CARDIO:	TIME	DISTANCE	PACE	HR

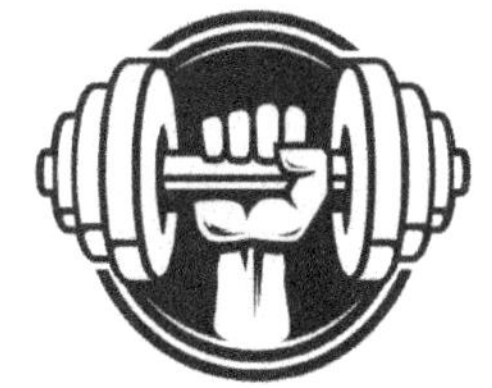

NAME:

DATE:

TIME START:

TIME END:

WARM-UP	TIME	NOTES

STRETCH:	TIME	NOTES

EXERCISE:	SET 1		SET 2		SET 3		SET 4	
	REPS	WEIGHT	REPS	WEIGHT	REPS	WEIGHT	REPS	WEIGHT

CARDIO:	TIME	DISTANCE	PACE	HR

NAME:

DATE:

TIME START:

TIME END:

WARM-UP	TIME	NOTES

STRETCH:	TIME	NOTES

EXERCISE:	SET 1		SET 2		SET 3		SET 4	
	REPS	WEIGHT	REPS	WEIGHT	REPS	WEIGHT	REPS	WEIGHT

CARDIO:	TIME	DISTANCE	PACE	HR

NAME: _________________________

DATE: _________________________

TIME START: ____________________

TIME END: ______________________

WARM-UP	TIME	NOTES

STRETCH:	TIME	NOTES

EXERCISE:	SET 1		SET 2		SET 3		SET 4	
	REPS	WEIGHT	REPS	WEIGHT	REPS	WEIGHT	REPS	WEIGHT

CARDIO:	TIME	DISTANCE	PACE	HR

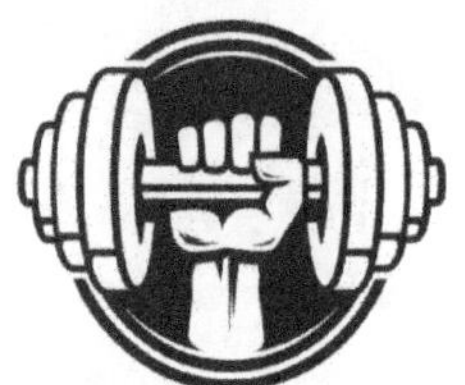

NAME: _______________________

DATE: _______________________

TIME START: _______________________

TIME END: _______________________

WARM-UP	TIME	NOTES

STRETCH:	TIME	NOTES

EXERCISE:	SET 1		SET 2		SET 3		SET 4	
	REPS	WEIGHT	REPS	WEIGHT	REPS	WEIGHT	REPS	WEIGHT

CARDIO:	TIME	DISTANCE	PACE	HR

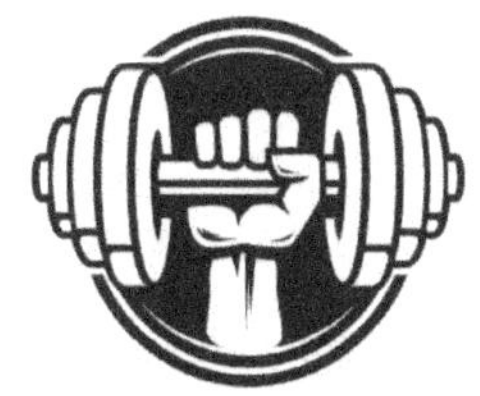

NAME:______________________

DATE:______________________

TIME START:______________________

TIME END:______________________

WARM-UP	TIME	NOTES

STRETCH:	TIME	NOTES

EXERCISE:	SET 1		SET 2		SET 3		SET 4	
	REPS	WEIGHT	REPS	WEIGHT	REPS	WEIGHT	REPS	WEIGHT

CARDIO:	TIME	DISTANCE	PACE	HR

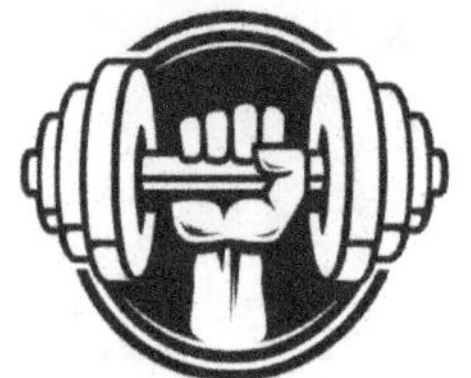

NAME: ______________________

DATE: ______________________

TIME START: ______________________

TIME END: ______________________

WARM-UP	TIME	NOTES

STRETCH:	TIME	NOTES

EXERCISE:	SET 1		SET 2		SET 3		SET 4	
	REPS	WEIGHT	REPS	WEIGHT	REPS	WEIGHT	REPS	WEIGHT

CARDIO:	TIME	DISTANCE	PACE	HR

NAME:

DATE:

TIME START:

TIME END:

WARM-UP	TIME	NOTES

STRETCH:	TIME	NOTES

EXERCISE:	SET 1		SET 2		SET 3		SET 4	
	REPS	WEIGHT	REPS	WEIGHT	REPS	WEIGHT	REPS	WEIGHT

CARDIO:	TIME	DISTANCE	PACE	HR

NAME:_________________________

DATE:_________________________

TIME START:_________________________

TIME END:_________________________

WARM-UP	TIME	NOTES

STRETCH:	TIME	NOTES

EXERCISE:	SET 1		SET 2		SET 3		SET 4	
	REPS	WEIGHT	REPS	WEIGHT	REPS	WEIGHT	REPS	WEIGHT

CARDIO:	TIME	DISTANCE	PACE	HR

NAME: \
DATE: \
TIME START: \
TIME END:

WARM-UP	TIME	NOTES

STRETCH:	TIME	NOTES

EXERCISE:	SET 1		SET 2		SET 3		SET 4	
	REPS	WEIGHT	REPS	WEIGHT	REPS	WEIGHT	REPS	WEIGHT

CARDIO:	TIME	DISTANCE	PACE	HR

NAME:

DATE:

TIME START:

TIME END:

WARM-UP	TIME	NOTES

STRETCH:	TIME	NOTES

EXERCISE:	SET 1		SET 2		SET 3		SET 4	
	REPS	WEIGHT	REPS	WEIGHT	REPS	WEIGHT	REPS	WEIGHT

CARDIO:	TIME	DISTANCE	PACE	HR

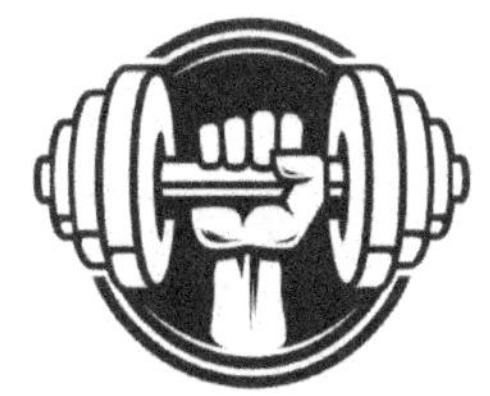

NAME: _______________________

DATE: _______________________

TIME START: _______________________

TIME END: _______________________

WARM-UP	TIME	NOTES

STRETCH:	TIME	NOTES

EXERCISE:	SET 1		SET 2		SET 3		SET 4	
	REPS	WEIGHT	REPS	WEIGHT	REPS	WEIGHT	REPS	WEIGHT

CARDIO:	TIME	DISTANCE	PACE	HR

NAME:_______________________

DATE:_______________________

TIME START:_______________________

TIME END:_______________________

WARM-UP	TIME	NOTES

STRETCH:	TIME	NOTES

EXERCISE:	SET 1		SET 2		SET 3		SET 4	
	REPS	WEIGHT	REPS	WEIGHT	REPS	WEIGHT	REPS	WEIGHT

CARDIO:	TIME	DISTANCE	PACE	HR

NAME: _______________________

DATE: _______________________

TIME START: _______________________

TIME END: _______________________

WARM-UP	TIME	NOTES

STRETCH:	TIME	NOTES

EXERCISE:	SET 1		SET 2		SET 3		SET 4	
	REPS	WEIGHT	REPS	WEIGHT	REPS	WEIGHT	REPS	WEIGHT

CARDIO:	TIME	DISTANCE	PACE	HR

NAME:

DATE:

TIME START:

TIME END:

WARM-UP	TIME	NOTES

STRETCH:	TIME	NOTES

EXERCISE:	SET 1		SET 2		SET 3		SET 4	
	REPS	WEIGHT	REPS	WEIGHT	REPS	WEIGHT	REPS	WEIGHT

CARDIO:	TIME	DISTANCE	PACE	HR

NAME:

DATE:

TIME START:

TIME END:

WARM-UP	TIME	NOTES

STRETCH:	TIME	NOTES

EXERCISE:	SET 1		SET 2		SET 3		SET 4	
	REPS	WEIGHT	REPS	WEIGHT	REPS	WEIGHT	REPS	WEIGHT

CARDIO:	TIME	DISTANCE	PACE	HR

NAME:

DATE:

TIME START:

TIME END:

WARM-UP	TIME	NOTES

STRETCH:	TIME	NOTES

EXERCISE:	SET 1		SET 2		SET 3		SET 4	
	REPS	WEIGHT	REPS	WEIGHT	REPS	WEIGHT	REPS	WEIGHT

CARDIO:	TIME	DISTANCE	PACE	HR

NAME: _______________________

DATE: _______________________

TIME START: _______________________

TIME END: _______________________

WARM-UP	TIME	NOTES

STRETCH:	TIME	NOTES

EXERCISE:	SET 1		SET 2		SET 3		SET 4	
	REPS	WEIGHT	REPS	WEIGHT	REPS	WEIGHT	REPS	WEIGHT

CARDIO:	TIME	DISTANCE	PACE	HR

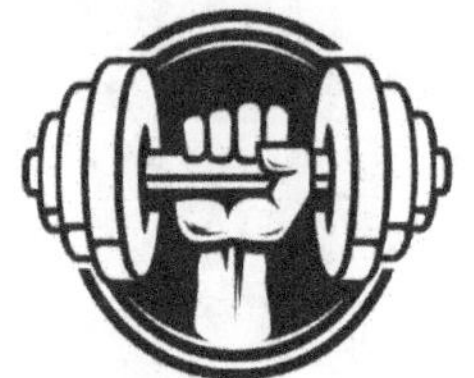

NAME:	
DATE:	
TIME START:	
TIME END:	

WARM-UP	TIME	NOTES

STRETCH:	TIME	NOTES

EXERCISE:	SET 1		SET 2		SET 3		SET 4	
	REPS	WEIGHT	REPS	WEIGHT	REPS	WEIGHT	REPS	WEIGHT

CARDIO:	TIME	DISTANCE	PACE	HR

NAME:

DATE:

TIME START:

TIME END:

WARM-UP	TIME	NOTES

STRETCH:	TIME	NOTES

EXERCISE:	SET 1		SET 2		SET 3		SET 4	
	REPS	WEIGHT	REPS	WEIGHT	REPS	WEIGHT	REPS	WEIGHT

CARDIO:	TIME	DISTANCE	PACE	HR

NAME:________________________

DATE:________________________

TIME START:________________________

TIME END:________________________

WARM-UP	TIME	NOTES

STRETCH:	TIME	NOTES

EXERCISE:	SET 1		SET 2		SET 3		SET 4	
	REPS	WEIGHT	REPS	WEIGHT	REPS	WEIGHT	REPS	WEIGHT

CARDIO:	TIME	DISTANCE	PACE	HR

NAME: ________________________

DATE: ________________________

TIME START: ________________________

TIME END: ________________________

WARM-UP	TIME	NOTES

STRETCH:	TIME	NOTES

EXERCISE:	SET 1		SET 2		SET 3		SET 4	
	REPS	WEIGHT	REPS	WEIGHT	REPS	WEIGHT	REPS	WEIGHT

CARDIO:	TIME	DISTANCE	PACE	HR

NAME:

DATE:

TIME START:

TIME END:

WARM-UP	TIME	NOTES

STRETCH:	TIME	NOTES

EXERCISE:	SET 1		SET 2		SET 3		SET 4	
	REPS	WEIGHT	REPS	WEIGHT	REPS	WEIGHT	REPS	WEIGHT

CARDIO:	TIME	DISTANCE	PACE	HR

NAME: _______________________

DATE: _______________________

TIME START: _______________________

TIME END: _______________________

WARM-UP	TIME	NOTES

STRETCH:	TIME	NOTES

EXERCISE:	SET 1		SET 2		SET 3		SET 4	
	REPS	WEIGHT	REPS	WEIGHT	REPS	WEIGHT	REPS	WEIGHT

CARDIO:	TIME	DISTANCE	PACE	HR

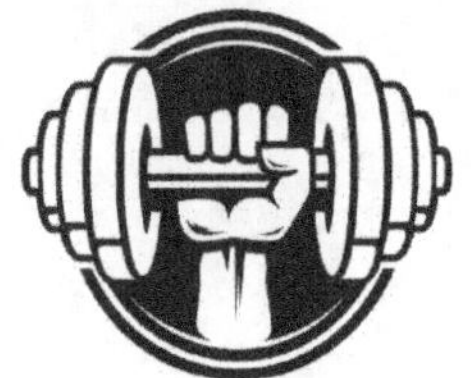

NAME:______________________

DATE:______________________

TIME START:______________________

TIME END:______________________

WARM-UP	TIME	NOTES

STRETCH:	TIME	NOTES

EXERCISE:	SET 1		SET 2		SET 3		SET 4	
	REPS	WEIGHT	REPS	WEIGHT	REPS	WEIGHT	REPS	WEIGHT

CARDIO:	TIME	DISTANCE	PACE	HR

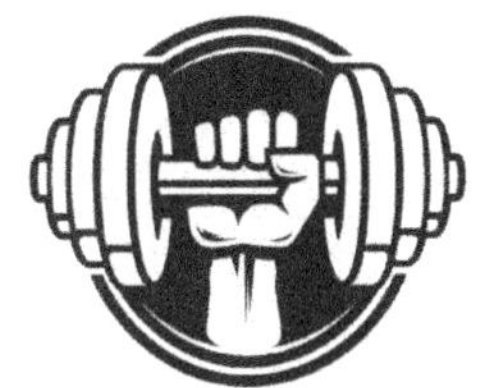

NAME:

DATE:

TIME START:

TIME END:

WARM-UP	TIME	NOTES

STRETCH:	TIME	NOTES

EXERCISE:	SET 1		SET 2		SET 3		SET 4	
	REPS	WEIGHT	REPS	WEIGHT	REPS	WEIGHT	REPS	WEIGHT

CARDIO:	TIME	DISTANCE	PACE	HR

NAME:________________________________

DATE:________________________________

TIME START:________________________________

TIME END:________________________________

WARM-UP	TIME	NOTES

STRETCH:	TIME	NOTES

EXERCISE:	SET 1		SET 2		SET 3		SET 4	
	REPS	WEIGHT	REPS	WEIGHT	REPS	WEIGHT	REPS	WEIGHT

CARDIO:	TIME	DISTANCE	PACE	HR